Copyright

H. QUINONES MD

All rights reserved. No part of this publication may be reproduced, distributed, or transmitted in any form or by any means, including photocopying, recording, or other electronic or mechanical methods, without the prior written permission of the publisher, except in the case of brief quotations embodied in critical reviews and certain other noncommercial uses permitted by copyright law.

Contents

- Introduction 5
- Notable trials on motor symptoms (tremor, slowness, stiffness): 6
- CBD Oil 9
  - Is CBD marijuana 9
  - Where does CBD come from 10
  - How CBD works 10
  - Benefits 11
  - Side effects 20
  - Risks 20
  - Side effects of Epidiolex 20
  - Side effects of other uses of CBD 21
  - How to use 22
- Parkinson's disease 24
  - Parkinson's definition and disease facts 25
  - Theory of PD Progression: Braak's Hypothesis 28
  - What are the early signs and symptoms of Parkinson's disease 29
  - What are the later secondary signs and symptoms of Parkinson's disease 30
  - Causes of Parkinson's disease 31
  - What are the 5 stages of Parkinson's disease 32
  - Is Parkinson's disease inherited (genetic) 33

Who gets Parkinson's disease	35
What tests diagnose Parkinson's disease	35
Diagnosis	36
Treatment	37
Medications	38
Lifestyle and home remedies	44
Alternative medicine	46
Coping and support	47
Preparing for your appointment	48
What you can do	48
Write down questions to ask your doctor	49
What to expect from your doctor	50
What is the treatment for Parkinson's disease	52
What is the prognosis and life expectancy for Parkinson's disease	54
Gut-brain axis	56
Mitochondria, microbiota and marijuana	58
Pot for Parkinson's	60
A threshold dose	62
Lifestyle Modifications for PD Patients	63
Can Parkinson's disease be prevented	65
What other conditions resemble Parkinson's disease	65
How can people learn to cope with Parkinson's disease	66

LEARNING HOW TO MANAGE DAILY LIVING WITH PARKINSON'S 67
CBD AND PARKINSON'S DISEASE 70
Cannabis and the brain 71
The Endocannabinoid System 72
Why Can CBD Work For Treating Parkinson's Disease 73
What Are The Benefits Of Using CBD To Treat Parkinson's Disease 74
The Endocannabinoid System & Parkinson's Disease 75
How Can I Use CBD To Treat Parkinson's Disease 76
What Are Studies Saying About Using CBD For Parkinson's Disease 77
Cannabinoids as neuroprotectants 78
best cbd oil for parkinson's 79
Marijuana and Public Health 80
THC and CBD 81
Clinical Trials in Parkinson's disease with CBD and THC 83
Medical Marijuana Availability 84
Tips and take-aways 86
Patients turn to cannabis 86
Clinical Trials for CBD and Parkinson's - Past and Future 87
Which CBD Oil Is Best For Parkinson's 88

Introduction

Parkinson's disease is a progressive nervous system disorder that affects movement. Symptoms start gradually, sometimes starting with a barely noticeable tremor in just one hand. Tremors are common, but the disorder also commonly causes stiffness or slowing of movement.

Our bodies make natural cannabinoids that control sleep, appetite, mood and other processes by binding to receptors throughout the body and brain. These receptors are found in particularly high numbers in the basal ganglia, a circuit of brain cells that controls movement and is affected in Parkinson's. Because the cannabinoids in marijuana bind to the receptors in our body and brain, researchers have looked at whether they could bind to basal ganglia and other receptors to modify the course of PD or help ease symptoms of disease.

Parkinson's disease (PD) can be very challenging to cope with, causing a mixture of motor and non-motor symptoms that affect nearly every aspect of daily living. Although the medications that doctors prescribe can be helpful, there remain gaps in what the medications can treat. Understandably, people with PD are eager to find alternative methods to help their symptoms, leading many of these patients to look into whether other therapies, such as medical marijuana, also known as medical cannabis, can be useful.

Pre-clinical work, including several studies funded by MJFF, shows that cannabinoids may protect brain cells through antioxidant and anti-inflammatory mechanisms.

Clinical studies have evaluated whether marijuana can ease Parkinson's motor and non-motor symptoms as well as levodopa-induced dyskinesia, involuntary movements that may result with long-term use of levodopa and many years of living with PD. In general, trials show mixed results (some positive, some negative), which leaves patients, doctors and researchers with insufficient evidence that medical marijuana and cannabinoids are an effective treatment for Parkinson's.

Notable trials on motor symptoms (tremor, slowness, stiffness):

A randomized, placebo-controlled, double-blind trial of two different doses of CBD capsules improved quality of life but not motor symptoms in 21 people with PD.

An open-label study of smoked marijuana decreased tremor and slowness in 22 people with PD.

For non-motor symptoms:

An open-label study of CBD tablets decreased psychosis -- hallucinations (seeing things that aren't there) and delusions (having false, often paranoid, beliefs) in six people with PD.

An open-label study of CBD tablets lessened symptoms of REM sleep behavior disorder (acting out dreams) in four people with Parkinson's.

Formal studies on other non-motor symptoms have not been conducted, but many individuals cite anecdotal benefit on pain, anxiety and sleep problems (as well as motor symptoms).

Noteworthy trials on levodopa-induced dyskinesia:

A randomized, placebo-controlled, double-blind trial of a capsule containing THC and CBD did not improve dyskinesia or motor symptoms in 17 people with Parkinson's.

A randomized, placebo-controlled, double-blind trial of nabilone (an FDA-approved man-made cannabinoid for chemotherapy-related nausea/vomiting and AIDS-related weight loss) improved dyskinesia in seven people with PD. In a randomized, placebo-controlled, double-blind trial, one group of participants receives the study drug while another receives placebo (an inactive substance that looks exactly like the study drug). Neither participant nor researcher knows who is getting study drug or placebo.

In an open-label study, there is no placebo group, and both participants and researchers know what treatment is being given.

In the early stages of Parkinson's disease, your face may show little or no expression. Your arms may not swing when you walk. Your speech may become soft or slurred. Parkinson's disease symptoms worsen as your condition progresses over time.

Although Parkinson's disease can't be cured, medications might significantly improve your symptoms. Occasionally, your doctor may suggest surgery to regulate certain regions of your brain and improve your symptoms.

CBD Oil

CBD is one of many compounds, known as cannabinoids, in the cannabis plant. Researchers have been looking at the possible therapeutic uses of CBD.

CBD oils are oils that contain concentrations of CBD. The concentrations and the uses of these oils vary.

Is CBD marijuana

- CBD oil may have a number of health benefits.
- Until recently, the best-known compound in cannabis was delta-9 tetrahydrocannabinol (THC).
- This is the most active ingredient in marijuana.
- Marijuana contains both THC and CBD, and these compounds have different effects.
- THC creates a mind-altering "high" when a person smokes it or uses it in cooking. This is because THC breaks down when we apply heat and introduce it into the body.
- CBD is different. Unlike THC, it is not psychoactive. This means that CBD does not change a person's state of mind when they use it.

However, CBD does appear to produce significant changes in the body, and some research suggests that it has medical benefits.

Where does CBD come from

The least processed form of the cannabis plant is hemp. Hemp contains most of the CBD that people use medicinally. Hemp and marijuana come from the same plant, Cannabis sativa, but the two are very different.

Over the years, marijuana farmers have selectively bred their plants to contain high levels of THC and other compounds that interested them, often because the compounds produced a smell or had another effect on the plant's flowers.

However, hemp farmers have rarely modified the plant. These hemp plants are used to create CBD oil.

How CBD works

All cannabinoids, including CBD, produce effects in the body by attaching to certain receptors.

The human body produces certain cannabinoids on its own. It also has two receptors for cannabinoids, called the CB1 receptors and CB2 receptors.

CB1 receptors are present throughout the body, but many are in the brain.

The CB1 receptors in the brain deal with coordination and movement, pain, emotions, and mood, thinking, appetite, and memories, and other functions. THC attaches to these receptors.

CB2 receptors are more common in the immune system. They affect inflammation and pain.

Researchers once believed that CBD attached to these CB2 receptors, but it now appears that CBD does not attach directly to either receptor. Instead, it seems to direct the body to use more of its own cannabinoids.

Benefits
- CBD may benefit a person's health in a variety of ways.
- Natural pain relief and anti-inflammatory properties
- People tend to use prescription or over-the-counter drugs to relieve stiffness and pain, including chronic pain.
- Some people believe that CBD offers a more natural alternative.
- Authors of a study published in the Journal of Experimental Medicine found that CBD

significantly reduced chronic inflammation and pain in some mice and rats.

- The researchers suggested that the non-psychoactive compounds in marijuana, such as CBD, could provide a new treatment for chronic pain.

Quitting smoking and drug withdrawals

Some promising evidence suggests that CBD use may help people to quit smoking.

A pilot study published in Addictive Behaviors found that smokers who used inhalers containing CBD smoked fewer cigarettes than usual and had no further cravings for nicotine.

A similar review, published in Neurotherapeutics found that CBD may be a promising treatment for people with opioid addiction disorders.

The researchers noted that CBD reduced some symptoms associated with substance use disorders. These included anxiety, mood-related symptoms, pain, and insomnia.

More research is necessary, but these findings suggest that CBD may help to prevent or reduce withdrawal symptoms.

Epilepsy

After researching the safety and effectiveness of CBD oil for treating epilepsy, the FDA approved the use of CBD (Epidiolex) as a therapy for two rare conditions characterized by epileptic seizures in 2018.

In the U.S., a doctor can prescribe Epidiolex to treat:

- Lennox-Gastaut syndrome (LGS), a condition that appears between the ages of 3 and 5 years and involves different kinds of seizures
- Dravet syndrome (DS), a rare genetic condition that appears in the first year of life and involves frequent, fever-related seizures

The types of seizures that characterize LGS or DS are difficult to control with other types of medication. The FDA specified that doctors could not prescribe Epidiolex for children younger than 2 years. A physician or pharmacist will determine the right dosage based on body weight.

Other neurological symptoms and disorders

Researchers are studying the effects of CBD on various neuropsychiatric disorders.

Authors of a 2014 review noted that CBD has anti-seizure properties and a low risk of side effects for people with epilepsy.

Findings suggested that CBD may also treat many complications linked to epilepsy, such as neurodegeneration, neuronal injury, and psychiatric diseases.

Another study, published in Current Pharmaceutical Design, found that CBD may produce effects similar to those of certain antipsychotic drugs, and that the compound may provide a safe and effective treatment for people with schizophrenia. However, further research is necessary.

Fighting cancer

Some researchers have found that CBD may prove to combat cancer.

Authors of a review published in the British Journal of Clinical Pharmacology found evidence that CBD significantly helped to prevent the spread of cancer.

The researchers also noted that the compound tends to suppress the growth of cancer cells and promote their destruction.

They pointed out that CBD has low levels of toxicity. They called for further research into its potential as an accompaniment to standard cancer treatments.

Anxiety disorders

Doctors often advise people with chronic anxiety to avoid cannabis, as THC can trigger or amplify feelings of anxiousness and paranoia. However, authors of a review from Neurotherapeutics found that CBD may help to reduce anxiety in people with certain related disorders.

According to the review, CBD may reduce anxiety-related behaviors in people with conditions such as:

- post-traumatic stress disorder
- general anxiety disorder
- panic disorder
- social anxiety disorder
- obsessive-compulsive disorder

The authors noted that current treatments for these disorders can lead to additional symptoms and side effects, which can cause some people to stop taking them.

No further definitive evidence currently links CBD to adverse effects, and the authors called for further studies of the compound as a treatment for anxiety.

Type 1 diabetes

Type 1 diabetes results from inflammation that occurs when the immune system attacks cells in the pancreas.

Research published in 2016 by Clinical Hemorheology and Microcirculation found that CBD may ease this inflammation in the pancreas. This may be the first step in finding a CBD-based treatment for type 1 diabetes.

A paper presented in the same year in Lisbon, Portugal, suggested that CBD may reduce inflammation and protect against or delay the development of type 1 diabetes.

Acne

Acne treatment is another promising use for CBD. The condition is caused, in part, by inflammation and overworked sebaceous glands in the body.

A 2014 study published by the Journal of Clinical Investigation found that CBD helps to lower the production of sebum that leads to acne, partly because of its anti-inflammatory effect on the body. Sebum is an oily substance, and overproduction can cause acne.

CBD could become a future treatment for acne vulgaris, the most common form of acne.

Alzheimer's disease

Initial research published in the Journal of Alzheimer's Disease found that CBD was able to prevent the development of social recognition deficit in participants.

This means that CBD could help people in the early stages of Alzheimer's to keep the ability to recognize the faces of people that they know.

This is the first evidence that CBD may slow the progression of Alzheimer's disease.

Legality

CBD oil is a cannabinoid derived from the cannabis plant.

Cannabis is legal for either medicinal or recreational use in some American states. Other states have approved the use of CBD oil as a hemp product but not the general use of medical marijuana.

Some state and federal laws differ, and current marijuana and CBD legislation in the U.S. can be confusing, even in states where marijuana is legal.

There is an ever-changing number of states that do not necessarily consider marijuana to be legal but have laws directly related to CBD oil. The following information is accurate as of May 8, 2018, but the laws change frequently.

However, state legislators generally approve the use of CBD oil at various concentrations to treat a range of epileptic conditions. A full list of states that have CBD-specific laws is available here.

Different states also require different levels of prescription to possess and use CBD oil. In Missouri, for example, a person can use CBD of a particular composition if they can show that three other treatment options have failed to treat their epilepsy.

Anyone considering CBD oil should speak with a local healthcare provider. They can provide information about safe CBD sources and local laws surrounding usage.

Recent developments: CBD oil for epilepsy

In June 2018, the FDA approved the use of CBD to treat two types of epilepsy.

Dr. Scott Gottlieb, writing for the FDA on 25 June, stated:

- "Today, the FDA approved a purified form of the drug cannabidiol (CBD). This is one of more than 80 active chemicals in marijuana. The new product was approved to treat seizures associated with two rare, severe forms of epilepsy in patients two years of age and older."

Dr. Gottlieb is careful to point out that:

- The FDA have not approved the use of marijuana or all of its components.
- The association has only approved a purified version of one CBD medication, for a precise therapeutic purpose.
- The decision to approve the product was based on the results of sound clinical trials.
- Patients will receive the medication in a reliable dosage.

Side effects

Many small-scale studies have looked into the safety of CBD in adults. They concluded that adults tend to tolerate a wide range of doses well.

Researchers have found no significant side effects on the central nervous system, the vital signs, or mood, even among people who used high dosages.

The most common side effect was tiredness. Also, some people reported diarrhea and changes in appetite or weight.

Risks

There is still a lack of available long-term safety data.

Also, to date, researchers have not performed studies involving children.

Side effects of Epidiolex

Concerning the product that the FDA approved to treat two types of epilepsy, researchers noticed following adverse effects in clinical trials:

- liver problems
- symptoms related to the central nervous system, such as irritability and lethargy
- reduced appetite

- gastrointestinal problems
- infections
- rashes and other sensitivity reactions
- reduced urination
- breathing problems

The patient information leaflet notes that there is a risk of worsening depression or suicidal thoughts. It is important to monitor anyone who is using this drug for signs of mood change.

Research suggests that a person taking the product is unlikely to form a dependency.

Side effects of other uses of CBD

There is often a lack of evidence regarding the safety of new or alternative treatment options. Usually, researchers have not performed the full array of tests.

Anyone who is considering using CBD should talk to a qualified healthcare practitioner beforehand.

The FDA have only approved CBD for the treatment of two rare and severe forms of epilepsy.

When drugs do not have FDA approval, it can be difficult to know whether a product contains a safe or effective level of CBD. Unapproved products may not have the properties or contents stated on the packaging.

It is important to note that researchers have linked marijuana use during pregnancy to impairments in the fetal development of neurons. Regular use among teens is associated with issues concerning memory, behavior, and intelligence.

How to use
CBD is one of the compounds in marijuana

CBD is just one of may compounds in marijuana, and it is not psychoactive. Smoking cannabis is not the same as using CBD oil.

Using CBD oil is not the same as using or smoking whole cannabis.

A person can use CBD oil in different ways to relieve various symptoms.

If a doctor prescribes it to treat LGS or DS, it is important to follow their instructions.

CBD-based products come in many forms. Some can be mixed into different foods or drinks or taken with a pipette or dropper.

Others are available in capsules or as a thick paste to be massaged into the skin. Some products are available as sprays to be administered under the tongue.

Recommended dosages vary between individuals, and depend on factors such as body weight, the concentration of the product, and the health issue.

Some people consider taking CBD oil to help treat:

- chronic pain
- epilepsy
- Parkinson's disease
- Huntington's disease
- sleep disorders
- glaucoma

Due to the lack of FDA regulation for most CBD products, seek advice from a medical professional before determining the best dosage.

As regulation in the U.S. increases, more specific dosages and prescriptions will start to emerge.

After discussing dosages and risks with a doctor, and researching regional local laws, it is important to compare different brands of CBD oil.

Parkinson's disease

Parkinson's disease is the second most common neurodegenerative disorder and the most common movement disorder. Characteristics of Parkinson's disease are progressive loss of muscle control, which leads to trembling of the limbs and head while at rest, stiffness, slowness, and impaired balance. As symptoms worsen, it may become difficult to walk, talk, and complete simple tasks.

The progression of Parkinson's disease and the degree of impairment vary from person to person. Many people with Parkinson's disease live long productive lives, whereas others become disabled much more quickly. Complications of Parkinson's such as falling-related injuries or pneumonia. However, studies of patent populations with and without Parkinson's Disease suggest the life expectancy for people with the disease is about the same as the general population.

Most people who develop Parkinson's disease are 60 years of age or older. Since overall life expectancy is rising, the number of individuals with Parkinson's disease will increase in the future. Adult-onset Parkinson's disease is most common, but early-onset Parkinson's disease (onset between 21-40 years), and juvenile-onset Parkinson's disease (onset before age 21) can occur.

Descriptions of Parkinson's disease date back as far as 5000 BC. Around that time, an ancient Indian civilization called the disorder Kampavata and treated it with the seeds of a plant containing therapeutic levels of what is today known as levodopa. Parkinson's disease was named after the British doctor James Parkinson, who in 1817 first described the disorder in detail as "shaking palsy."

Parkinson's definition and disease facts

Parkinson's disease is a neurodegenerative disorder, which leads to progressive deterioration of motor function due to loss of dopamine-producing brain cells.

The cause of Parkinson's Disease is unknown but researchers speculate that both genetic and environmental factors are involved; some genes have been linked to the disease.

Primary symptoms include:

- Tremor
- Stiffness
- Slowness
- Impaired balance
- Shuffling gait later in the disease

Some secondary symptoms include:

- Anxiety
- Depression
- Dementia

Most people with Parkinson's disease are diagnosed when they are 60 years old or older, but early-onset Parkinson's disease also occurs.

Several staging systems for Parkinson's disease exist. The Parkinson's Disease Foundation supports 5 stages, which include:

- Stage 1. Symptoms are mild and do not interfere with the person's quality of life.
- Stage 2. Symptoms worsen and daily activities become more difficult and take more time to complete.
- Stage 3 is considered mid-stage Parkinson's disease. The individual loses balance, moves more slowly, and falls are common. Symptoms impair daily activities, for example, dressing, eating, and brushing teeth.
- Stage 4. Symptoms become severe and the individual needs assistance walking and performing daily activities.
- Stage 5 is the most advanced stage of Parkinson's disease. The individual is unable to walk and will need full time assistance with living.

With proper treatment, most individuals with Parkinson's disease can lead long, productive lives. The life expectancy is about the same as people without the disease.

Rating Scales

- Your doctor may refer to a scale to help them understand the progression of the disease. Parkinson's stages correspond both to the severity of movement symptoms and to how much the disease affects a person's daily activities. The most commonly used rating scales focus on motor symptoms. They are the: Hoehn and Yahr stages follow a simple rating scale, first introduced in 1967. Clinicians use it to describe how motor symptoms progress in PD.
- Rates symptoms on a scale of 1 to 5. On this scale, 1 and 2 represent early-stage, 2 and 3 mid-stage, and 4 and 5 advanced-stage Parkinson's.
- The Unified Parkinson's Disease Rating Scale (UPDRS) is a more comprehensive tool used to account for non-motor symptoms, including mental functioning, mood and social interaction.

- Accounts for cognitive difficulties, ability to carry out daily activities and treatment complications.
- New scales include information on non-motor symptoms (such as sense of smell).

While symptoms and disease progression are unique to each person, knowing the typical stages of Parkinson's can help you cope with changes as they occur. Some people experience the changes over 20 years or more. Others find the disease progresses more quickly.

Theory of PD Progression: Braak's Hypothesis

The current theory (part of the so-called Braak's hypothesis) is that the earliest signs of Parkinson's are found in the enteric nervous system, the medulla and the olfactory bulb, which controls sense of smell. Under this theory, Parkinson's only progresses to the substantia nigra and cortex over time. This theory is increasingly borne out by evidence that non-motor symptoms, such as a loss of sense of smell (hyposmia), sleep disorders and constipation may precede the motor features of the disease by several years. For this reason, researchers are increasingly focused on these non-motor symptoms to detect PD as early as possible and to look for ways to stop its progression.

What are the early signs and symptoms of Parkinson's disease

The primary symptoms of Parkinson's disease are all related to voluntary and involuntary motor function and usually start on one side of the body. Symptoms are mild at first and will progress over time. Some people are more affected than others are. Studies have shown that by the time that primary symptoms appear, individuals with Parkinson's disease will have lost 60% to 80% or more of the dopamine-producing cells in the brain. Characteristic motor symptoms include:

- Tremors: Trembling in fingers, hands, arms, feet, legs, jaw, or head. Usually tremors occur while resting, but not while involved in a task. Tremors may worsen when a person is excited, tired, or stressed.
- Rigidity: Stiffness of the limbs and trunk, which may increase during movement. Rigidity may produce muscle aches and pain. Loss of fine hand movements can lead to cramped handwriting (micrographia) and may make eating difficult.
- Bradykinesia: Slowness of voluntary movement. Over time, it may become difficult to initiate movement and to complete

movement. Bradykinesia together with stiffness can also affect the facial muscles and result in an expressionless, "mask-like" appearance.
- Postural instability: Impaired or lost reflexes can make it difficult to adjust posture to maintain balance. Postural instability may lead to falls.
- Parkinsonian gait: Individuals with more progressive Parkinson's disease develop a distinctive shuffling walk with a stooped position and a diminished or absent arm swing. It may become difficult to start walking and to make turns. Individuals may freeze in mid-stride and appear to fall forward while walking.

What are the later secondary signs and symptoms of Parkinson's disease

While the main symptoms of Parkinson's disease are movement-related, progressive loss of muscle control and continued damage to the brain can lead to secondary symptoms. These secondary symptoms vary in severity, and not everyone with Parkinson's will experience all of them, and may include:

- Anxiety, insecurity, and stress
- Confusion
- Memory loss
- Dementia (more common in the elderly)

- Constipation
- Depression
- Difficulty swallowing and excessive salivation
- Diminished sense of smell
- Increased sweating
- Erectile dysfunction (ED)
- Skin problems
- Slowed, quieter speech, and monotone voice
- Urinary frequency/urgency

Causes of Parkinson's disease

A substance called dopamine acts as a messenger between two brain areas - the substantia nigra and the corpus striatum - to produce smooth, controlled movements. Most of the movement-related symptoms of Parkinson's disease are caused by a lack of dopamine due to the loss of dopamine-producing cells in the substantia nigra. When the amount of dopamine is too low, communication between the substantia nigra and corpus striatum becomes ineffective, and movement becomes impaired; the greater the loss of dopamine, the worse the movement-related symptoms. Other cells in the brain also degenerate to some degree and may contribute to non-movement related symptoms of Parkinson's disease.

Although it is well known that lack of dopamine causes the motor symptoms of Parkinson's disease, it is not clear why the dopamine-producing brain cells deteriorate. Genetic and pathological studies have revealed that various dysfunctional cellular processes, inflammation, and stress can all contribute to cell damage. In addition, abnormal clumps called Lewy bodies, which contain the protein alpha-synuclein, are found in many brain cells of individuals with Parkinson's disease. The function of these clumps in regards to Parkinson's disease is not understood. In general, scientists suspect that dopamine loss is due to a combination of genetic and environmental factors.

What are the 5 stages of Parkinson's disease

Researchers may disagree on the number of stages of Parkinson's disease (range from 3-5 stages). However, they all agree the disease is a progressive disease with symptoms that usually occur in one stage may overlap or occur in another stage. The stage increase in number value for all stage naming systems reflect the increasing severity of the disease. The five stages used by the Parkinson's Foundation are:

- Stage 1: mild symptoms (tremors and/or movement symptoms like swinging arm while

walking) do not interfere with daily activities and occur on one side of the body.
- Stage 2: Symptoms worsen with walking problems and both sides of the body affected.
- Stage 3: Main symptoms worsen with loss of balance and slowness of movement.
- Stage 4: Severity of symptoms require help; usually person cannot live alone.
- Stage 5: Caregiver needed for all activities; patient may not be able to stand or walk and may be bedridden and may also experience hallucinations and delusions.

Is Parkinson's disease inherited (genetic)

In most people with Parkinson's disease is idiopathic, which means that it arises sporadically with no known cause. However, some of people diagnosed with Parkinson's also have family members with the disease. By studying families with hereditary Parkinson's disease, scientists have identified several genes that are associated with the disorder. Studying these genes helps understand the cause of Parkinson's disease and may lead to new therapies. So far, five genes have been identified that are definitively associated with Parkinson's disease.

- SNCA (synuclein, alpha non A4 component of amyloid precursor): SNCA makes the protein alpha-synuclein. In brain cells of individuals with Parkinson's disease, this protein aggregates in clumps called Lewy bodies. Mutations in the SNCA gene are found in early-onset Parkinson's disease.

- PARK2 (Parkinson's disease autosomal recessive, juvenile 2): The PARK2 gene makes the protein parkin. Mutations of the PARK2 gene are mostly found in individuals with juvenile Parkinson's disease. Parkin normally helps cells break down and recycle proteins.
- PARK7 (Parkinson's disease autosomal recessive, early onset 7): PARK7 mutations are found in early-onset Parkinson's disease. The PARK7 gene makes the DJ-1 protein, which may protect cells from oxidative stress.
- PINK1 (PTEN-induced putative kinase 1): Mutations of this gene are found in early-onset Parkinson's disease. The exact function of the protein made by PINK1 is not known, but it may protect structures within the cell called mitochondria from stress.
- LRRK2 (leucine-rich repeat kinase 2): LRRK2 makes the protein dardarin. Mutations in the LRRK2 gene have been linked to late-onset Parkinson's disease.

Several other chromosome regions and the genes GBA (glucosidase beta acid), SNCAIP (synuclein alpha interacting protein), and UCHL1 (ubiquitin carboxyl-terminal esterase L1) may also be linked to Parkinson's disease.

Who gets Parkinson's disease
- Age is the largest risk factor for the development and progression of Parkinson's disease. Most people who develop Parkinson's disease are older than 60 years of age.
- Men are affected about 1.5 to 2 times more often than women.
- A small number of individuals are at increased risk because of a family history of the disorder.
- Head trauma, illness, or exposure to environmental toxins such as pesticides and herbicides may be a risk factor.

What tests diagnose Parkinson's disease
An early and accurate diagnosis of Parkinson's disease is important in developing good treatment strategies to maintain a high quality of life for as long as possible. However, there is no test to diagnose Parkinson's disease with certainty (except after the individual has passed away). A diagnosis of Parkinson's disease - especially in the early phase - can be challenging due to similarities to related

movement disorders and other conditions with Parkinson-like symptoms. Individuals may sometimes be misdiagnosed as having another disorder, and sometimes individuals with Parkinson-like symptoms may be inaccurately diagnosed as having Parkinson's disease. It is therefore important to re-evaluate individuals in the early phase on a regular basis to rule out other conditions that may be responsible for the symptoms.

Diagnosis

No specific test exists to diagnose Parkinson's disease. Your doctor trained in nervous system conditions (neurologist) will diagnose Parkinson's disease based on your medical history, a review of your signs and symptoms, and a neurological and physical examination. Your doctor may suggest a specific single-photon emission computerized tomography SPECT scan called a dopamine transporter (DAT) scan. Although this can help support the suspicion that you have Parkinson's disease, it is your symptoms and neurologic examination that ultimately determine the correct diagnosis. Most people do not require a DAT scan.

Your doctor may order lab tests, such as blood tests, to rule out other conditions that may be causing your symptoms.

Imaging tests — such as MRI, CT, ultrasound of the brain, and PET scans — may also be used to help rule out other disorders. Imaging tests aren't particularly helpful for diagnosing Parkinson's disease.

In addition to your examination, your doctor may give you carbidopa-levodopa (Rytary, Sinemet, others), a Parkinson's disease medication. You must be given a sufficient dose to show the benefit, as low doses for a day or two aren't reliable. Significant improvement with this medication will often confirm your diagnosis of Parkinson's disease.

Sometimes it takes time to diagnose Parkinson's disease. Doctors may recommend regular follow-up appointments with neurologists trained in movement disorders to evaluate your condition and symptoms over time and diagnose Parkinson's disease.

Treatment

Parkinson's disease can't be cured, but medications can help control your symptoms, often dramatically. In some later cases, surgery may be advised.

Your doctor may also recommend lifestyle changes, especially ongoing aerobic exercise. In some cases, physical therapy that focuses on balance and stretching also is important. A speech-language pathologist may help improve your speech problems.

Medications

Medications may help you manage problems with walking, movement and tremor. These medications increase or substitute for dopamine.

People with Parkinson's disease have low brain dopamine concentrations. However, dopamine can't be given directly, as it can't enter your brain.

You may have significant improvement of your symptoms after beginning Parkinson's disease treatment. Over time, however, the benefits of drugs frequently diminish or become less consistent. You can usually still control your symptoms fairly well.

Medications your doctor may prescribe include:

- Carbidopa-levodopa. Levodopa, the most effective Parkinson's disease medication, is a natural chemical that passes into your brain and is converted to dopamine.
- Levodopa is combined with carbidopa (Lodosyn), which protects levodopa from early conversion to dopamine outside your brain. This prevents or lessens side effects such as nausea.

Side effects may include nausea or lightheadedness (orthostatic hypotension).

After years, as your disease progresses, the benefit from levodopa may become less stable, with a tendency to wax and wane ("wearing off").

Also, you may experience involuntary movements (dyskinesia) after taking higher doses of levodopa. Your doctor may lessen your dose or adjust the times of your doses to control these effects.

Carbidopa-levodopa infusion. Duopa is a brand-name medication made up of carbidopa and levodopa. However, it's administered through a feeding tube that delivers the medication in a gel form directly to the small intestine.

Duopa is for patients with more-advanced Parkinson's who still respond to carbidopa-levodopa, but who have a lot of fluctuations in their response. Because Duopa is continually infused, blood levels of the two drugs remain constant.

Placement of the tube requires a small surgical procedure. Risks associated with having the tube include the tube falling out or infections at the infusion site.

Dopamine agonists. Unlike levodopa, dopamine agonists don't change into dopamine. Instead, they mimic dopamine effects in your brain.

They aren't as effective as levodopa in treating your symptoms. However, they last longer and may be used with levodopa to smooth the sometimes off-and-on effect of levodopa.

Dopamine agonists include pramipexole (Mirapex), ropinirole (Requip) and rotigotine (Neupro, given as a patch). Apomorphine (Apokyn), is a short-acting injectable dopamine agonist used for quick relief.

Some of the side effects of dopamine agonists are similar to the side effects of carbidopa-levodopa. But they can also include hallucinations, sleepiness and compulsive behaviors such as hypersexuality, gambling and eating. If you're taking these medications and you behave in a way that's out of character for you, talk to your doctor.

MAO B inhibitors. These medications include selegiline (Eldepryl, Zelapar), rasagiline (Azilect) and safinamide (Xadago). They help prevent the breakdown of brain dopamine by inhibiting the brain enzyme monoamine oxidase B (MAO B). This enzyme metabolizes brain dopamine. Side effects may include nausea or insomnia.

When added to carbidopa-levodopa, these medications increase the risk of hallucinations.

These medications are not often used in combination with most antidepressants or certain narcotics due to potentially serious but rare reactions. Check with your doctor before taking any additional medications with an MAO B inhibitor.

Catechol O-methyltransferase (COMT) inhibitors. Entacapone (Comtan) is the primary medication from this class. This medication mildly prolongs the effect of levodopa therapy by blocking an enzyme that breaks down dopamine.

Side effects, including an increased risk of involuntary movements (dyskinesia), mainly result from an enhanced levodopa effect. Other side effects include diarrhea or other enhanced levodopa side effects.

Tolcapone (Tasmar) is another COMT inhibitor that is rarely prescribed due to a risk of serious liver damage and liver failure.

Anticholinergics. These medications were used for many years to help control the tremor associated with Parkinson's disease. Several anticholinergic medications are available, including benztropine (Cogentin) or trihexyphenidyl.

However, their modest benefits are often offset by side effects such as impaired memory, confusion, hallucinations, constipation, dry mouth and impaired urination.

Amantadine. Doctors may prescribe amantadine alone to provide short-term relief of symptoms of mild, early-stage Parkinson's disease. It may also be given with carbidopa-levodopa therapy during the later stages of Parkinson's disease to control involuntary movements (dyskinesia) induced by carbidopa-levodopa.

Side effects may include a purple mottling of the skin, ankle swelling or hallucinations.

- Surgical procedures
- Electrode placement and device location in deep brain stimulation

Deep brain stimulation

Deep brain stimulation. In deep brain stimulation (DBS), surgeons implant electrodes into a specific part of your brain. The electrodes are connected to a generator implanted in your chest near your collarbone that sends electrical pulses to your brain and may reduce your Parkinson's disease symptoms.

Your doctor may adjust your settings as necessary to treat your condition. Surgery involves risks, including infections, stroke or brain hemorrhage. Some people experience problems with the DBS system or have complications due to stimulation, and your doctor may need to adjust or replace some parts of the system.

Deep brain stimulation is most often offered to people with advanced Parkinson's disease who have unstable medication (levodopa) responses. DBS can stabilize medication fluctuations, reduce or halt involuntary movements (dyskinesia), reduce tremor, reduce rigidity, and improve slowing of movement.

DBS is effective in controlling erratic and fluctuating responses to levodopa or for controlling dyskinesia that doesn't improve with medication adjustments.

However, DBS isn't helpful for problems that don't respond to levodopa therapy apart from tremor. A tremor may be controlled by DBS even if the tremor isn't very responsive to levodopa.

Although DBS may provide sustained benefit for Parkinson's symptoms, it doesn't keep Parkinson's disease from progressing.

Lifestyle and home remedies

If you've received a diagnosis of Parkinson's disease, you'll need to work closely with your doctor to find a treatment plan that offers you the greatest relief from symptoms with the fewest side effects. Certain lifestyle changes also may help make living with Parkinson's disease easier.

Healthy eating

While no food or combination of foods has been proved to help in Parkinson's disease, some foods may help ease some of the symptoms. For example, eating foods high in fiber and drinking an adequate amount of fluids can help prevent constipation that is common in Parkinson's disease.

A balanced diet also provides nutrients, such as omega-3 fatty acids, that might be beneficial for people with Parkinson's disease.

Exercise

Exercising may increase your muscle strength, flexibility and balance. Exercise can also improve your well-being and reduce depression or anxiety.

Your doctor may suggest you work with a physical therapist to learn an exercise program that works for you. You may also try exercises such as walking, swimming, gardening, dancing, water aerobics or stretching.

Parkinson's disease can disturb your sense of balance, making it difficult to walk with a normal gait. Exercise may improve your balance. These suggestions may also help:

- Try not to move too quickly.
- Aim for your heel to strike the floor first when you're walking.
- If you notice yourself shuffling, stop and check your posture. It's best to stand up straight.
- Look in front of you, not directly down, while walking.
- Avoiding falls

In the later stages of the disease, you may fall more easily. In fact, you may be thrown off balance by just a small push or bump. The following suggestions may help:

- Make a U-turn instead of pivoting your body over your feet.
- Distribute your weight evenly between both feet, and don't lean.
- Avoid carrying things while you walk.
- Avoid walking backward.
- Daily living activities

Daily living activities — such as dressing, eating, bathing and writing — can be difficult for people with Parkinson's disease. An occupational therapist can show you techniques that make daily life easier.

Alternative medicine

Supportive therapies can help ease some of the symptoms and complications of Parkinson's disease, such as pain, fatigue and depression. When performed in combination with your treatments, these therapies might improve your quality of life:

- Massage. Massage therapy can reduce muscle tension and promote relaxation. This therapy, however, is rarely covered by health insurance.
- Tai chi. An ancient form of Chinese exercise, tai chi employs slow, flowing motions that may improve flexibility, balance and muscle strength. Tai chi may also prevent falls. Several forms of tai chi are tailored for people of any age or physical condition.

A study showed tai chi may improve the balance of people with mild to moderate Parkinson's disease more than stretching and resistance training.

- Yoga. In yoga, gentle stretching movements and poses may increase your flexibility and

balance. You may modify most poses to fit your physical abilities.
- Alexander technique. This technique — which focuses on muscle posture, balance and thinking about how you use muscles — may reduce muscle tension and pain.
- Meditation. In meditation, you quietly reflect and focus your mind on an idea or image. Meditation may reduce stress and pain and improve your sense of well-being.
- Pet therapy. Having a dog or cat may increase your flexibility and movement and improve your emotional health.

Coping and support

Living with any chronic illness can be difficult, and it's normal to feel angry, depressed or discouraged at times. Parkinson's disease, in particular, can be profoundly frustrating, as walking, talking and even eating become more difficult and time-consuming.

Depression is common in people with Parkinson's disease. But antidepressant medications can help ease the symptoms of depression, so talk with your doctor if you're feeling persistently sad or hopeless.

Although friends and family can be your best allies, the understanding of people who know what you're going through can be especially helpful. Support groups aren't for everyone. However, for many people with Parkinson's disease and their families, a support group can be a good resource for practical information about Parkinson's disease.

Also, groups offer a place for you to find people who are going through similar situations and can support you.

You and your family may also benefit from talking to a mental health professional, such as a psychologist or social worker trained in working with people who have chronic conditions.

Preparing for your appointment

You're likely to first see your primary care doctor. However, you may then be referred to a doctor trained in nervous system disorders (neurologist).

Because there's often a lot to discuss, it's a good idea to prepare for your appointment. Here's some information to help you get ready for your appointment and what to expect from your doctor.

What you can do
- Write down any symptoms you're experiencing, including any that may seem unrelated to the

reason for which you scheduled the appointment.
- Write down key personal information, including any major stresses or recent life changes.
- Make a list of all medications, vitamins and supplements that you're taking.
- Ask a family member or friend to come with you, if possible. Sometimes it can be difficult to remember all of the information provided to you during an appointment. Someone who accompanies you may remember something that you missed or forgot.

Write down questions to ask your doctor.
Your time with your doctor is limited, so preparing a list of questions ahead of time will help you make the most of your time together. For Parkinson's disease, some basic questions to ask your doctor include:

- What's the most likely cause of my symptoms?
- Are there other possible causes?
- What kinds of tests do I need? Do these tests require any special preparation?
- How does Parkinson's disease usually progress?
- Will I eventually need long-term care?
- What treatments are available, and which do you recommend for me?

- What types of side effects can I expect from treatment?
- If the treatment doesn't work or stops working, do I have additional options?
- I have other health conditions. How can I best manage these conditions together?
- Are there any brochures or other printed material that I can take home with me? What websites do you recommend?

In addition to the questions that you've prepared to ask your doctor, don't hesitate to ask questions that occur to you during your appointment.

What to expect from your doctor

Your doctor is likely to ask you a number of questions. Being ready to answer them may reserve time to go over any points you want to spend more time on. Your doctor may ask:

- When did you first begin experiencing symptoms?
- Do you have symptoms all the time or do they come and go?
- Does anything seem to improve your symptoms?
- Does anything seem to make your symptoms worse?

A neurologist who specializes in movement disorders will be able to make the most accurate diagnosis. An initial assessment is made based on medical history, a neurological exam, and the symptoms present. For the medical history, it is important to know whether other family members have Parkinson's disease, what types of medication have been or are being taken, and whether there was exposure to toxins or repeated head trauma previously. A neurological exam may include an evaluation of coordination, walking, and fine motor tasks involving the hands.

Several guidelines have been published to assist in the diagnosis of Parkinson's disease. These include the Hoehn and Yahr scale and the Unified Parkinson's Disease Rating Scale. Tests are used to measure mental capacity, behavior, mood, daily living activities, and motor function. They can be very helpful in the initial diagnosis, to rule out other disorders, as well as in monitoring the progression of the disease to make therapeutic adjustments. Brain scans and other laboratory tests are also sometimes carried out, mostly to detect other disorders resembling Parkinson's disease.

The diagnosis of Parkinson's disease is more likely if:

- At least two of the three major symptoms are present (tremor at rest, muscle rigidity, and slowness)

- The onset of symptoms started on one side of the body
- Symptoms are not due to secondary causes such as medication or strokes in the area controlling movement
- Symptoms are significantly improved with levodopa

What is the treatment for Parkinson's disease

There is currently no treatment to cure Parkinson's disease. Several therapies are available to delay the onset of motor symptoms and to ameliorate motor symptoms. All of these therapies are designed to increase the amount of dopamine in the brain either by replacing dopamine, mimicking dopamine, or prolonging the effect of dopamine by inhibiting its breakdown. Studies have shown that early therapy in the non-motor stage can delay the onset of motor symptoms, thereby extending quality of life.

The most effective therapy for Parkinson's disease is levodopa (Sinemet), which is converted to dopamine in the brain. However, because long-term treatment with levodopa can lead to unpleasant side effects (a shortened response to each dose, painful cramps, and involuntary movements), its use is often delayed until motor impairment is more severe. Levodopa is frequently prescribed together with carbidopa

(Sinemet), which prevents levodopa from being broken down before it reaches the brain. Co-treatment with carbidopa allows for a lower levodopa dose, thereby reducing side effects.

In earlier stages of Parkinson's disease, substances that mimic the action of dopamine (dopamine agonists), and substances that reduce the breakdown of dopamine (monoamine oxidase type B (MAO-B) inhibitors) can be very efficacious in relieving motor symptoms. Unpleasant side effects of these preparations are quite common, including swelling caused by fluid accumulation in body tissues, drowsiness, constipation, dizziness, hallucinations, and nausea.

For some individuals with advanced, virtually unmanageable motor symptoms, surgery may be an option. In deep brain stimulation (DBS), the surgeon implants electrodes to stimulate areas of the brain involved in movement. In another type of surgery, specific areas in the brain that cause Parkinson's symptoms are destroyed.

An alternative approach that has been explored is the use of dopamine-producing cells derived from stem cells. While stem cell therapy has great potential, more research is required before such cells can become of therapeutic value in the treatment of Parkinson's disease.

In addition to medication and surgery, general lifestyle changes (rest and exercise), physical therapy, occupational therapy, and speech therapy may be beneficial.

What is the prognosis and life expectancy for Parkinson's disease

The severity of Parkinson's disease symptoms and signs vary greatly from person to peson, and it is not possible to predict how quickly the disease will progress. Parkinson's disease itself is not a fatal disease, and the average life expectancy is similar to that of people without the disease. Secondary complications, such as pneumonia, falling-related injuries, and choking can lead to death. Many treatment options can reduce some of the symptoms and prolong the quality of life.

Dopamine depletion

Parkinson's Disease is most associated with compromised motor function after the loss of 60-80% of dopamine-producing neurons. As dopaminergic neurons become damaged or die and the brain is less able to produce adequate amounts of dopamine, patients may experience any one or combination of these classic PD motor symptoms: tremor of the hands, arms, legs or jaw; muscle rigidity or stiffness of the limbs and trunk; slowness of movement (bradykinesia); and /or impaired balance and coordination (postural instability).

Additional symptoms include decreased facial expressions, dementia or confusion, fatigue, sleep disturbances, depression, constipation, cognitive changes, fear, anxiety, and urinary problems. Pesticide exposure and traumatic brain injury are linked to increased risk for PD. Paraquat, an herbicide sprayed by the DEA in anti-marijuana defoliant operations in the United States and other countries, resembles a toxicant MPTP [methyl-phenyl-tetrahydropyridien], which is used to simulate animal models of Parkinson's for research purposes.

Within the PD brain there are an inordinate number of Lewy bodies - intracellular aggregates of difficult to break down protein clusters - that cause dysfunction and demise of neurons.(3) This pathological process results in difficulties with thinking, movement, mood and behavior. The excessive presence of Lewy bodies, coupled with the deterioration of dopaminergic neurons, are considered to be hallmarks of Parkinson's. But mounting evidence suggests that these aberrations are actually advanced-stage manifestations of a slowly evolving pathology.

It appears that non-motor symptoms occur for years before the disease progresses to the brain, and that PD is actually a multi-system disorder, not just a neurological ailment, which develops over a long period of time. According to the National Parkinson's Foundation, motor symptoms of PD only begin to manifest when most of the brain's dopamine-producing cells are already damaged.

Patients whose PD is diagnosed at an early stage have a better chance of slowing disease progression. The most common approach to treating PD is with oral intake of L-dopa, the chemical precursor to dopamine. But in some patients, long-term use of L-dopa will exacerbate PD symptoms. Unfortunately, there is no cure – yet.

Gut-brain axis

What causes Parkinson's? One theory that is gaining favor among medical scientists traces the earliest signs of PD to the enteric nervous system (the gut), the medulla (the brainstem), and the olfactory bulb in the brain, which controls one's sense of smell. New research shows that the quality of bacteria in the gut the microbiome is strongly implicated in the advancement of Parkinson's, the severity of symptoms, and related mitochondrial dysfunction.

Defined as "the collection of all the microorganisms living in association with the human body," the microbiome consists of "a variety of microorganisms including eukaryotes, archaea, bacteria and viruses." Bacteria, both good and bad, influence mood, gut motility, and brain health. There is a strong connection between the microbiome and the endocannabinoid system: Gut microbiota modulate intestinal endocannabinoid tone, and endocannabinoid signaling mediates communication between the central and the enteric nervous systems, which comprise the gut-brain axis.

Viewed as "the second brain," the enteric nervous system consists of a mesh-like web of neurons that covers the lining of the digestive tract from mouth to anus and everything in between. The enteric nervous system generates neurotransmitters and nutrients, sends signals to the brain, and regulates gastrointestinal activity. It also plays a major role in inflammation.

The mix of microorganisms that inhabit the gut and the integrity of the gut lining are fundamental to overall health and the ability of the gut-brain axis to function properly. If the lining of the gut is weak or unhealthy, it becomes more permeable and allows things to get into the blood supply that should not be there, negatively impacting the immune system. This is referred to as "leaky gut." Factor in an overgrowth of harmful bacteria and a paucity of beneficial bacteria and you have a recipe for a health disaster.

The importance of a beneficial bacteria in the gut and a well-balanced microbiome cannot be overstated. Bacterial overgrowth in the small intestine, for example, has been associated with worsening PD motor function. In a 2017 article in the European Journal of Pharmacology, titled "The gut-brain axis in Parkinson's disease: Possibilities for food-based therapies," Peres-Pardo et al examine the interplay between gut dysbiosis and Parkinson's. The authors note that "PD pathogenesis may be caused or exacerbated by dysbiotic microbiota-induced inflammatory responses ... in the intestine and the brain."

Mitochondria, microbiota and marijuana

The microbiome also plays an important role in the health of our mitochondria, which are present in every cell in the brain and body (except red blood cells). Mitochondria function not only as the cell's power plant; they also are involved in regulating cell repair and cell death. Dysfunction of the mitochondria, resulting in high levels of oxidative stress, is intrinsic to PD neurodegeneration. Microbes produce inflammatory chemicals in the gut that seep into the bloodstream and damage mitochondria, contributing to disease pathogenesis not only in PD but many neurological and metabolic disorders, including obesity, type-2 diabetes, and Alzheimer's.

The evidence that gut dysbiosis can foster the development of PD raises the possibility that those with the disease could benefit by manipulating their intestinal bacteria and improving their microbiome. Enhancing one's diet with fermented foods and probiotic supplements may improve gut health and relieve constipation, while also reducing anxiety, depression and memory problems that afflict PD patients.

Cannabis therapeutics may also help to manage PD symptoms and slow the progression of the disease. Acclaimed neurologist Sir William Gowers was the first to mention cannabis as a treatment for tremors in 1888. In his Manual of Diseases of the Nervous System, Grower noted that oral consumption of an "Indian hemp" extract quieted tremors temporarily, and after a year of chronic use the patient's tremors nearly ceased.

Modern scientific research supports the notion that cannabis could be beneficial in reducing inflammation and assuaging symptoms of PD, as well as mitigating disease progression to a degree. Federally-funded preclinical probes have documented the robust antioxidant and neuroprotective properties of CBD and THC with "particular application ... in the treatment of neurodegenerative diseases, such as Alzheimer's disease, Parkinson's disease and HIV dementia." Published in 1998, these findings formed the basis of a U.S. government patent on cannabinoids as antioxidants and neuroprotectants.

Pot for Parkinson's

Although clinical studies focusing specifically on the use of plant cannabinoids to treat PD are limited (because of marijuana prohibition) and convey conflicting results, in aggregate they provide insight into how cannabis may aid those with Parkinson's. Cannabidiol, THC, and especially THCV all showed sufficient therapeutic promise for PD in preclinical studies to warrant further investigation. Additional research might shed light on which plant cannabinoids, or combination thereof, is most appropriate for different stages of Parkinson's.

Anecdotal accounts from PD patients using artisanal cannabis preparations indicate that cannabinoid acids (present in unheated whole plant cannabis products) may reduce PD tremor and other motor symptoms. Raw cannabinoid acids (such as CBDA and THCA) are the chemical precursors to neutral, "activated" cannabinoids (CBD, THC). Cannabinoid acids become neutral cannabinoid compounds through a process called decarboxylation, where they lose their carboxyl group through aging or heat. Minimal research has focused on cannabinoid acids, but the evidence thus far suggests that THCA and CBDA have powerful therapeutic attributes, including anti-inflammatory, anti-nausea, anti-cancer, and anti-seizure properties. In a 2004 survey of cannabis use among patients at the Prague Movement Disorder Centre in the Czech Republic, 45 percent of respondents reported improvement in PD motor symptoms.

Cannabis clinicians are finding that dosage regimens for medical marijuana patients with PD don't conform to a one-size-fits-all approach. In her book Cannabis Revealed (2016), Dr. Bonni Goldstein discussed how varied a PD patient's response to cannabis and cannabis therapeutics can be:

- "A number of my patients with PD have reported the benefits of using different methods of delivery and different cannabinoid profiles. Some patients have found relief of tremors with inhaled THC and other have not. A few patients have found relief with high doses of CBD-rich cannabis taken sublingually. Some patients are using a combination of CBD and THC ... Trial and error is needed to find what cannabinoid profile and method will work best. Starting a low-dose and titrating up is

recommended, particularly with THC-rich cannabis. Unfortunately, THCV-rich varieties are not readily available."
- 0.5 g of smoked cannabis resulted in significant improvement in tremor and bradykinesia as well as sleep.
- 150 mg of CBD oil titrated up over four weeks resulted in decreased psychotic symptoms.
- 75-300 mg of oral CBD improved REM-behavior sleep disorder.

A threshold dose

Of course, each patient is different, and cannabis therapeutics is personalized medicine. Generally speaking, an optimal therapeutic combination will include a synergistic mix of varying amounts of CBD and THC – although PD patients with sleep disturbances may benefit from a higher THC ratio at night.

Dr. Russo offers cogent advice for patients with PD and other chronic conditions who are considering cannabis therapy. "In general," he suggests, "2.5 mg of THC is a threshold dose for most patients without prior tolerance to its effects, while 5 mg is a dose that may be clinically effective at a single administration and is generally acceptable, and 10 mg is a prominent dose, that may be too high for naïve and even some experienced subjects. These figures may be revised upward slightly if the preparation contains significant CBD content ... It is always advisable to start at a very low dose and titrate upwards slowly."

Lifestyle Modifications for PD Patients

It is important to treat the patient as a whole mind, body and soul. The following are a few lifestyle modifications that may provide relief from PD symptoms and improve quality of life.

- Do cardio aerobic exercise: This benefits the body in so many ways, including stimulating the production of one's endocannabinoids, increasing oxygen in the blood supply, mitigating the negative impact of oxidative stress, and boosting the production of BDNF, a brain-protecting chemical found to be low in PD patients.
- Eat more fruits and vegetables: The old saying "garbage in, garbage out" is so true. The majority of PD patients suffer from chronic constipation. A high fiber diet can be helpful in improving gut motility and facilitating daily bowel movements.
- Get restful sleep: Not getting good sleep can undermine one's immune function, cognition

and quality of life. The importance of adequate restful sleep cannot be over emphasized.
- Reduce protein intake – This may help reduce the accumulation of protein bodies that result in Lewy bodies that appear in the enteric nervous system and the central nervous system and increase the uptake of L-dopa.
- Practice meditation, yoga or Tai Chi: The focus on the integration of movement and breath not only improve mobility but it also improves cognition and immunity. One study showed an increase in grey matter density in the areas of the brain associated with PD. Another showed that yoga improved balance, flexibility, posture and gait in PD patients. Research shows that tai chi can improve balance, gait, functional mobility, and overall well being.
- Consume probiotic food and supplements: Probiotic foods — raw garlic, raw onions, bananas, asparagus, yams, sauerkraut, etc.— are a great source for the good bacteria in your large intestine. Augmenting your diet with probiotic supplements, especially after taking antibiotics, can support the immune system by helping to repopulate the upper digestive tract with beneficial bacteria. Consult your doctor regarding a recommendation for a quality probiotic.

- Drink coffee: The risk of PD is considerably lower for men who consume coffee daily.

Can Parkinson's disease be prevented

Scientists currently believe that Parkinson's disease is triggered through a complex combination of genetic susceptibility and exposure to environmental factors such as toxins, illness, and trauma. Since the exact causes are not known, Parkinson's disease is at present not preventable.

What other conditions resemble Parkinson's disease

In its early stages, Parkinson's disease can resemble a number of other conditions with Parkinson-like symptoms known as Parkinsonism. These conditions include:

- Multiple system atrophy
- Progressive supranuclear palsy
- Corticobasal degeneration,
- Lewy body dementia
- Stroke
- Encephalitis (inflammation of the brain)
- Head trauma

Alzheimer's disease and primary lateral sclerosis can also be mistaken for Parkinson's disease. Other similar conditions include essential tremor, dystonic tremor, vascular Parkinsonism, and drug-induced Parkinsonism.

How can people learn to cope with Parkinson's disease

Although Parkinson's disease progresses slowly, it will eventually affect every aspect of life - from social engagements, work, to basic routines. Accepting the gradual loss of independence can be difficult. Being well informed about the disease can reduce anxiety about what lies ahead. Many support groups offer valuable information for individuals with Parkinson's disease and their families on how to cope with the disorder. Local groups can provide emotional support as well as advice on where to find experienced doctors, therapists, and related information. It is also very important to stay in close contact with health care professionals to monitor the progression of the disease and to adjust therapies to maintain the highest quality of living.

LEARNING HOW TO MANAGE DAILY LIVING WITH PARKINSON'S

Once you are diagnosed with PD, your focus should be on improving your symptoms and maintaining an active and positive lifestyle.

Although there is currently no cure for PD, it is possible to successfully manage symptoms through healthy choices, medications, and, in select cases, medical procedures.

Exercise

Starting or continuing a schedule of regular exercise can make a big difference in your mobility, both in the short and long term. People with Parkinson's disease also report the physical (and mental) benefits of swimming, cycling, dancing, and even non-contact boxing. In fact, several research studies have shown that regular exercise routines of walking, strength training, or Tai Chi can help to maintain, or even improve, mobility, balance, and coordination in people with PD.

Diet

There is no one diet that is recommended for PD, but healthy eating in general is always a good choice. For example, eating several servings of fruits and vegetables a day increases fiber intake and can help alleviate constipation, in addition to promoting general health. Also, drinking plenty of water or other non-alcoholic and caffeine-free beverages ensures adequate hydration and may reduce the likelihood of muscle cramping. Also, fruits and vegetables high in antioxidants, such as blueberries, spinach, and green tea, may also be beneficial to your diet.

Medications

Although there is no cure for PD, there are several classes of medications available for the successful treatment of motor symptoms throughout the course of the disease. Be sure to talk with your general neurologist or movement disorder specialist about your most troubling symptoms and your goals for medical therapy. Some medications for Parkinson's disease are available in generic forms or through special programs, so that they are more affordable.

Assembling a capable health care team

Developing and maintaining relationships with experts in the field of Parkinson's disease can make life easier and more enjoyable. Your team members and the role or roles they assume are likely to change as your symptoms change and as the disease progresses. Some will go the distance, staying with you throughout your life with Parkinson's. Others will be sprinters, accompanying you as you manage particular symptoms, emotions, or transitions. Your team can include:

- Movement Disorder Specialist (a neurologist who specializes in Parkinson's disease)
- Nurse
- Physical Therapist
- Occupational Therapist
- Speech Therapist
- Social Worker
- Pharmacist
- Neuropsychologist
- Neurosurgeon
- Parkinson's Disease and Palliative Care

CBD AND PARKINSON'S DISEASE

The endocannabinoid system and digestive imbalance play major roles in Parkinson's disease. Research on CBD, THC, and THCV has demonstrated that cannabis medicine may help to manage PD symptoms. CBD activates a G-coupled protein receptor called "GPR6" that is highly expressed in the basal ganglia region of the brain. GPR6 is considered an "orphan receptor" because researchers have yet to find the primary endogenous compound that binds to this receptor. It has been shown that a depletion of GPR6 causes an increase of dopamine, a critical neurotransmitter, in the brain. This finding suggests GPR6 could have a role in the treatment of Parkinson's, a chronic, neurodegenerative disease that entails the progressive loss of dopaminergic (dopamine-producing) neurons and consequent impairment of motor control. By acting as an "inverse agonist" at the GPR6 receptor, CBD boosts dopamine levels in preclinical studies.

Parkinson's affects an estimated 10 million people worldwide, including one million Americans. It is the second most common neurological disorder (after Alzheimer's Disease). Over 96 percent of those diagnosed with PD are over 50 years old with men being one-and-a-half times more likely to have PD than women. Uncontrolled PD significantly reduces the patient's quality of life and can render a person unable to care for themselves, trapped in a body they cannot control.

Cannabis and the brain

Cannabis is a genus of plant that when ingested by humans, can exert numerous effects on the brain and body. The cannabis plant, of course, did not evolve to be used by humans. Humans however, are naturally curious about their environment, and discovered these effects nevertheless. In this regard, cannabis is no different from many other plants from which humans have extracted products, such as the foxglove plant from which digoxin, a medication for heart disease was derived, or the Taxus species of plants from which paclitaxel, a medication for certain cancers was derived.

With further scientific investigation, it was discovered that the effects of the cannabis plant occur through the binding of certain chemicals in cannabis to a system of receptors in the human brain, named the endocannabinoid system (ECS). Cannabis contains more than 60 of these chemicals.

The Endocannabinoid System

One of the key roles of the endocannabinoid system (ECS) is regulating the lifespan of a cell, something vitally important in the central nervous system where brain cell loss is particularly difficult to overcome. Scientists have come to realise that in neurodegenerative disease, the ECS may even have a neuroprotective effect, as indicated by alterations in endocannabinoid levels and receptor expression. While these ECS changes are open to interpretation, the conclusion reached is that they reflect the body trying to mitigate against the neuronal damage occurring as a result of the disease.

The area of the brain affected by Parkinson's, the basal ganglia, has a high density of CB1 receptors and in experimental Parkinson's models scientists have observed increased CB1 activity in this brain region. Greater CB2 receptor expression has also been noted in the brain's glial cells, as well as an overall increase in endocannabinoid production.

Researchers have already seen that botanical cannabinoids found in the cannabis plant can have a direct impact on the endocannabinoid system. It's no surprise then that an exciting area of research into combating neurodegenerative disease is the use of cannabinoids as therapeutic tools.

The endocannabinoid system (ECS) is composed of:

- receptors that are expressed throughout the nervous system
- ligands, which are natural chemicals manufactured in the body that bind to these receptors

Through this binding, the ECS regulates many functions including mood, pain, memory, and appetite. The name of this system is unfortunate, as it implies that it evolved with cannabis in mind. The reverse is true. First the ECS evolved in humans. Then scientists discovered that certain chemicals in the cannabis plant could mimic the naturally occurring chemicals that are meant to bind the receptors.

Why Can CBD Work For Treating Parkinson's Disease

The idea of CBD for treating or managing Parkinson's disease is still new to many people. However, the latest evidence shows that CBD can actually treat some of the symptoms associated with Parkinson's disease, like sleep disturbances, psychosis, and impaired movement.

CBD is extracted from cannabis and made into an oil. The hemp plant has Cannabidiol and Tetrahydrocannabinol (THC) as its two major components. CBD oil is extracted from hemp plants with a high concentration of Cannabidiol and very low concentration of its psychoactive cousin THC. This is why CBD is very effective in treatment without it being psychoactive.

The Endocannabinoid system in our bodies fights against our outer body state by maintaining an inner balance thus regulating our mood, appetite, temperature etc. The main cannabinoid receptors located throughout the body are called CB1 and CB2. CBD oil, when bonded to these receptors, helps the brain in producing more dopamine which is known to inhibit the symptoms of Parkinson's disease.

A study conducted in 2017 showed that CBD blocks a receptor known as GPR6 which is known to cause some impaired movements in a patient with Parkinson's. Another study showed positive results and improved quality of life for patients with the disease without any other psychiatric disorder.

What Are The Benefits Of Using CBD To Treat Parkinson's Disease

CBD is gaining popularity with time in the wellness and health world. Scientists confirm that it may be able to help different ailments like pain and anxiety.

Some of the benefits of using CBD to treat Parkinson's disease include:

- Improved Sleep
- Decreased Psychosis
- Anti-Inflammatory
- Neuroprotectant

Parkinsons is a neurodegenerative disease. CBD acts significantly as a neuroprotectant. It also acts as a powerful antioxidant. Oxidative stress is also believed to be a cause of Parkinson's disease.

The Endocannabinoid System & Parkinson's Disease

The Endocannabinoid System is a very important modulatory system in the immune tissues as well as the endocrine, and brain functions. It plays a major role in secreting hormones that are related to the body's response to stress and its reproductive functions. The two important receptors of this system are known as CB1 and CB2.

This system is known to modulate a big range of our bodies' physiological functions. These include motor control, pain, mood, feeding behavior, and cognition. Parkinson's disease affects most of these bodily functions. This means it directly affects the endocannabinoid system. In order for a patient to be able to manage the symptoms associated with Parkinson's disease, like the lack of motor functions, pain, interrupted sleep, etc., the endocannabinoid system should always perform at its peak, failure to which the patient will experience the symptoms and this will make their life hard to manage and control. The use of CBD helps to improve the receptors in the system which in turn will increase the overall functionality of the endocannabinoid system.

How Can I Use CBD To Treat Parkinson's Disease

You can incorporate CBD in your exercise to lessen the sensation of pain. Another way to use CBD in your recovery is by taking it after a long day. CBD oil can be used as a cream or lotion. You can apply it to relieve pain on part of the body and as a nerve relief.

A few drops of CBD oil ingested helps in controlling the shaking and tremors and even slowed movements.

Whether you are using CBD oil as a first timer or if you are an experienced user, it is important to follow the right dosage for treatment. Start small and increase gradually according to your symptoms and as directed by the physician.

CBD capsules are also available for use for individuals with Parkinson disease, follow the correct dosage and consult with your doctor on how it is working for you. Remember everyone is different so the reaction will differ from person to person even if the symptoms are the same. Therefore, start slowly and see how your body responds to the CBD oil.

To take CBD oil orally, hold it under the tongue for a few seconds before you swallow it. Other oral ways you can take CBD oil is in edibles like chocolate bars, chewing gum, or even mouth strips.

What Are Studies Saying About Using CBD For Parkinson's Disease

Over the years, studies have shown that early diagnosis of Parkinson's disease can lead to a better management of it over time. Researchers have continued to develop new kinds of treatments for those suffering from Parkinson's Disease. Some of the recent treatment areas being studied include gene therapy, the use of stem cells and fetal cell transplantation. Research has so far made some remarkable progress. Scientists now say that there is hope that the cause whether environmental or generic, will be identified and their effects on the functionality of the brain are understood.

Cannabinoids as neuroprotectants

While current Parkinson's medication seeks to redress the depletion of dopamine, the main focus of current cannabinoid research is into the neuroprotective, antioxidant and anti-inflammatory properties of the plant. Even the US Federal Government has patented cannabinoids as neuroprotectants and antioxidants for the treatment of diseases of the central nervous system.

cbd oil for parkinson's

THC, the most abundantly found cannabinoid in cannabis, binds perfectly with the CB1 receptor, eliciting a neuroprotective effect.

However, despite some favourable preclinical studies showing the THC's ability to reduce Parkinson's related excitotoxicity, scientists now know that CB1 activation can actually worsen the motor symptoms associated with the disease, thus taking THC out of the running.

But, all is not lost, because other cannabinoids also have a uniquely multi-pronged approach to protecting our brain cells both through ECS receptor activation, but also non-endocannabinoid system mechanisms.

And this is where CBD Oil for Parkinson's comes to the fore.

CBD and Parkinson's - how much do we know

CBD is generally a tricky cannabinoid to understand as it has poor binding affinity with endocannabinoid receptors. Much of its pharmacological effect comes from its interaction with other non-ECS receptors, as well as inhibiting the enzyme that metabolizes a key endocannabinoid in the body.

When it comes to CBD and Parkinson's, the compound has also been shown to block CB1 receptor activity, making it of particular interest for Parkinson's research.

best cbd oil for parkinson's
But it's as a powerful antioxidant that CBD shows most promise for Parkinson's. CBD scavenges the free radicals that cause oxidative stress, commonly believed to be a precursor to Parkinson's. Unlike other cannabinoids, it does so independently of any endocannabinoid signalling.

In the paper, 'Endocannabinoids and Neurodegenerative Disorders: Parkinson's Disease, Huntington's Chorea, Alzheimer's Disease, and

Others', the authors describe how "CBD is no less active against the brain damage produced by altered glutamate homeostasis than CBs that do target the CB1 receptor or those targeting the CB2 receptor against local inflammatory events."

Also of key importance is CBD's anti-inflammatory action, which again occurs independently of the endocannabinoid system, and is most likely related to the nuclear receptors of the PPAR family.

Marijuana and Public Health

Cannabis is a substance that can be abused – that is, taken for non-medical reasons in a manner that can be harmful. Cannabis can stimulate the reward system of the brain and cause a pleasurable "high", which can then be sought after by the user, leading to further use. Cannabis can change how a person perceives their surroundings and affect memory, reaction time, judgement, and ability to learn. Despite this, it was noted anecdotally by users that certain medical problems, such as chronic pain for example, were improved with marijuana. This led to efforts to create medical marijuana – purified chemicals from the cannabis plant, used at the doses that produce the desired result without harmful effects.

THC and CBD

The two primary chemicals that are isolated from the cannabis plant are Delta-9-tetrahydrocannibinol (THC) and Cannabidiol (CBD). THC exerts the mind-altering effects that recreational marijuana is known for, whereas CBD does not. For the most part, medical marijuana consists of purified combinations of these two chemicals in varying ratios. The combination can be dispensed as a liquid, pill or nasal spray. Both THC and CBD interact with the ECS.

Medical Marijuana and Parkinson's disease

Since CBD and THC are chemicals that occur naturally in a plant, they were by definition not designed to combat any of the symptoms of PD. It is unreasonable therefore to expect that they will be a solution to all that ails a person with Parkinson's. More research needs to be done, but based on what is known about the biology of cannabis, one could hypothesize that THC and/or CBD may be helpful for aspects of PD such as tremor, stiffness, insomnia, dystonia, pain, dyskinesias or weight loss. However, clinical trials are needed to prove:

- Which of these specific symptoms are helped?
- What ratios of THC and CBD work for a particular symptom?
- What doses of THC and CBD work for a particular symptom?

Because the history and politics of marijuana trigger such strong emotions, it is understandable that the public has begun to think of THC and CBD as unique substances with their own rules. But they should not be viewed this way. They are chemicals found in plants that have effects on the human brain and body and may help humans cope with some difficult medical symptoms. And if they are used by humans to cope with a medical symptom, then they are medications. To that end, we need to treat THC and CBD as the medications that they are and subject them to the same standards that we do any medication. Clinical trials can help us understand what symptoms they treat and what doses are needed. A major limitation to performing clinical trials with medical marijuana is that the federal government continues to consider marijuana an illegal substance and will not fund research involving marijuana. There are various efforts to try to change this, with the hope of opening up medical marijuana to further study. One must also consider that just like any medication, medical marijuana can interact with other prescription medications such as those that cause sleepiness or thin the blood. In addition, medical marijuana can have side effects. And just like any medication, the side effects will vary depending on the person taking it. Elderly patients are typically more susceptible to side effects, for example. Some side effects that might occur include sleepiness, confusion, difficulty concentrating, apathy, mood changes and gait imbalance. Therefore, before even considering medical marijuana, especially in the elderly, patients need to discuss how marijuana interacts with their other medications and weigh all the risks and benefits with their doctor.

Clinical Trials in Parkinson's disease with CBD and THC

A few clinical trials have been conducted investigating the role of CBD and THC in PD. In one, an open label study of CBD (in which doctor and patient were both aware that the patient was receiving treatment and there was no control group) was conducted on six patients with psychosis. Psychotic symptoms decreased. In a second trial, an open label study of CBD was conducted on four patients with REM behavior sleep disorder. Symptoms decreased. In a third, a double blinded trial of 21 patients were treated with CBD. Motor scores did not improve, but quality of life scores did. In another, patients at a movement disorders center were asked to fill out an anonymous questionnaire about their experience with cannabis. Of the 84 patients who admitted to using cannabis, 39 described mild or substantial improvement of PD symptoms including tremor and dyskinesias.

In 2017, the National Academies of Science, Engineering and Medicine released a report based on a review of 10,000 scientific abstracts concerning research into marijuana's effects on all aspects of health and disease. They published their conclusions. They concluded that there was not enough evidence in the literature to currently support the use of medical marijuana in PD as opposed to conditions such as chronic pain, chemotherapy-induced nausea, and multiple sclerosis among others, for which supportive evidence is available. This means that more studies need to be done in PD. One study is currently underway at University of Colorado.

Despite this lack of data, PD is typically one of the diseases for which a patient can obtain medical marijuana in the states in which it is available. Now the medical community needs to play catch up – and after the fact, provide the data to decide whether these medications truly work for symptoms of PD and are safe.

Medical Marijuana Availability

In the United States, medical marijuana is available in some form in 46 states, as well as Guam, Puerto Rico and the District of Columbia. However, there are vast differences between the states as to how the medical marijuana is regulated.

- In nine of those states, no doctor's recommendation is needed and marijuana is available for purchase by all adults.
- In 20 other states, medical marijuana products are available via a doctor's prescription.
- In 17 others, only CBD and low THC products are allowed to be dispensed with a doctor's prescription.
- In the remaining four states, there are no medical marijuana provisions. Marijuana in any form remains illegal from the federal government's perspective.
- In the states that require a doctor's prescription for medical marijuana, it is usually distributed from specific dispensaries and not from a general pharmacy. Doctors often are required to take a special course before they are allowed to prescribe. Many doctors have not taken this course which means that only a subset of doctors can prescribe marijuana. This leaves the ability to obtain medical marijuana highly variable from state to state. In some states, a person can purchase any product that he/she wants. In other states, a person needs to see a specific doctor (often not his/her own) to obtain the medical marijuana. And in other states, a person can't obtain medical marijuana at all.

Tips and take-aways

Discuss the decision of whether to try medical marijuana with your physician. Discuss whether you have particular symptoms that may be amenable to treatment with medical marijuana. Discuss whether you take any medications that could interact with medical marijuana and whether you might be at lower or higher risk for adverse side effects from medical marijuana.

If you try medical marijuana, assess the positive benefits and the side effects just like you would any medication that you try and report back to your physician.

Keep on the lookout for additional clinical trials to help assess whether medical marijuana is useful for specific PD symptoms.

Patients turn to cannabis

It's little wonder then that Parkinson's sufferers and their families, desperate to slow down the course of the disease and ameliorate the life limiting symptoms, look towards other options. And while, to some, cannabis might seem like a medical wildcard, its use for the disease can be traced back to the 19th Century, where it was described in William Richard

Gowers's "Manual of Diseases of the Nervous System."

Back then, very little was known about the chemical compounds in the plant.

Indeed, it's only in the last twenty years that scientists have really begun to understand how cannabis affects the body with the discovery of the endocannabinoid system the homeostatic regulator comprising a network of receptors (CB1 and CB2) and cannabis-like chemicals, found predominantly in the brain, central nervous and immune system.

Clinical Trials for CBD and Parkinson's - Past and Future

Until now there have been very few human studies examining CBD for Parkinson's.

One study, found CBD aided eye movement sleep behavior disorder, a condition commonly experienced by those with Parkinson's. However, in a 2014 double-blind trial in which 119 patients were given either a placebo, 75mg of CBD or 300mg of CBD, no significant changes were noted in motor symptoms or neuroprotective effects, although those taking 300mg CBD did report improvements in their quality of life.

Perhaps the most complete clinical study looking at CBD oil for Parkinson's is currently recruiting at the University of Colorado School of Medicine. Maureen Leehey MD will be using the GW Pharma CBD extract Epidiolex in a stage 1, open label trial to test its safety and tolerability.

A second stage crossover, double-blind, randomized controlled trial (RCT) should follow with 50 subjects testing whether CBD not only helps with tremors, but also improves anxiety and psychosis, cognition, anxiety, sleep, daytime sleepiness, mood, fatigue, pain, impulsivity, restless legs syndrome, and REM sleep behaviour disorder.

Which CBD Oil Is Best For Parkinson's

Though we cannot give you any specific advice about which of our products are best for Parkinson's Disease, we can guide you towards purchasing the best quality CBD oil.

Key to your decision should be finding CBD oils that are extracted from organic hemp, using state-of-the-art Supercritical CO_2 methods. This ensures you that the CBD oil is both free from solvents and that the active compounds like cannabinoids and terpenes are preserved.

But don't take our word for it. Always ask to see lab reports corresponding to the CBD oil you want to buy. It's the only way to know just how much CBD you are getting and to guarantee that there are no nasty chemicals, heavy metals or mold in the product.

At Endoca, we pride ourselves on controlling our production process from seed to shelf. Through our organic and Good Manufacturing Practice (GMP) certified production, we openly demonstrate our commitment towards customer satisfaction and safety.

Why not check out our TrustPilot Page, where you will find honest reviews about the quality of our products and customer service.

While it's still early days in the field of researching CBD Oil for Parkinson's, early results look promising. And as more clinical trials take place, perhaps science will eventually catch up with what many patients have already experienced firsthand.

Made in the USA
Las Vegas, NV
24 November 2023

81438118R00049